DEDICATION

I dedicate this book to my loving husband, if not for him I may not be able to live my life that way it is now. I may not have a perfect life but I know perfectly that this is the life that I want to have

TABLE OF CONTENTS

How to Beat Chronic Fatigue: What You Didn't Know

A Guide to Be Smart on Managing Fatigue

By: Deborah Adams

9781634289955

PUBLISHERS NOTES

Disclaimer – Speedy Publishing LLC

This publication is intended to provide helpful and informative material. It is not intended to diagnose, treat, cure, or prevent any health problem or condition, nor is intended to replace the advice of a physician. No action should be taken solely on the contents of this book. Always consult your physician or qualified health-care professional on any matters regarding your health and before adopting any suggestions in this book or drawing inferences from it.

The author and publisher specifically disclaim all responsibility for any liability, loss or risk, personal or otherwise, which is incurred as a consequence, directly or indirectly, from the use or application of any contents of this book.

Any and all product names referenced within this book are the trademarks of their respective owners. None of these owners have sponsored, authorized, endorsed, or approved this book.

Always read all information provided by the manufacturers' product labels before using their products. The author and publisher are not responsible for claims made by manufacturers.

This book was originally printed before 2014. This is an adapted reprint by Speedy Publishing LLC with newly updated content designed to help readers with much more accurate and timely information and data.

Speedy Publishing LLC

40 E Main Street, Newark, Delaware, 19711

Contact Us: 1-888-248-4521

Website: http://www.speedypublishing.co

REPRINTED Paperback Edition: ISBN: 9781634289955

Manufactured in the United States of America

Chapter 1 - A Short Overview

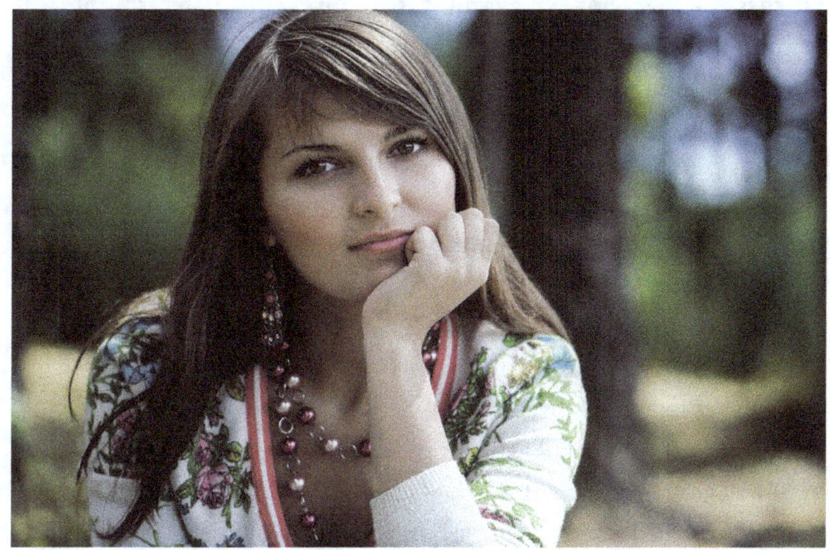

In sleep, all the voluntary muscles remain inactive and involuntary muscles functions are reduced. In other words, it is like switching off a machine or placing it in idle mode to allow the machines to cool off and prevent damage. It is mostly done at night where hormone levels are at the lowest.

How Sleep Works

A person's sleep can be affected by a lot of factors one of these factors include the circadian rhythm. The sleep-wake homeostasis or the circadian clock controls the sleep timing. It may have the greatest significance and greatest effect on the sleep of an individual. Sleep timing means the time you sleep and the time you wake up.

The circadian clock is also an inner time keeper, temperature controller, and an enzyme regulator. It is the rhythm that determines the ideal time for a person's restorative sleep and rest. It works together with a neurotransmitter called Adenosine.

Adenosine is a neurotransmitter responsible for inhibiting bodily processes involving wakefulness. Our circadian rhythm is commonly affected by poor sleeping habits such as overnight shifts, shifting time zones like flying from one country to another,

When a person goes to bed to rest, he or she undergoes a bodily and organized process called sleep. An individual passes through five phases of sleep: stages 1, 2, 3, 4, and REM (Rapid Eye Movement).

These stages progress into a cycle from stage 1 to REM. The cycle may be repeated more than twice in one night. An individual spends about 50% of his sleeping time in stage 2 of the cycle, 20% in REM and 30% is spent on the other part of the cycle. Infants on the other hand have different percentages wherein they spend about half of their sleeping time in REM.

Stage 1 is the stage in between sleep and wakefulness. A person's sleep would be easily disrupted if the person is in this stage. Muscle activity is still constant and the eye movements are still observed.

For the stage 2, the person's sleep gradually deepens. It is harder to wake a person in this stage of sleep.

On stages 3 and 4, a person no longer responds to environmental stimuli, Stimuli include loud noises and bright lights. It is the stage where the person stays before progressing to REM.

REM or Rapid Eye movement is part of the sleeping stage which a person enters approximately 90 minutes after sleep is initiated. The deepest stage in the sleep cycle and is the hardest time to wake up a person.

Muscle activity is greatly reduced but the brain activity is noticeably highest. EEG tests confirm that a person's brain activity during the REM stage is similar to that when a person is awake.

Chapter 2- Beat Chronic Fatigue - Take the Much Needed Sleep

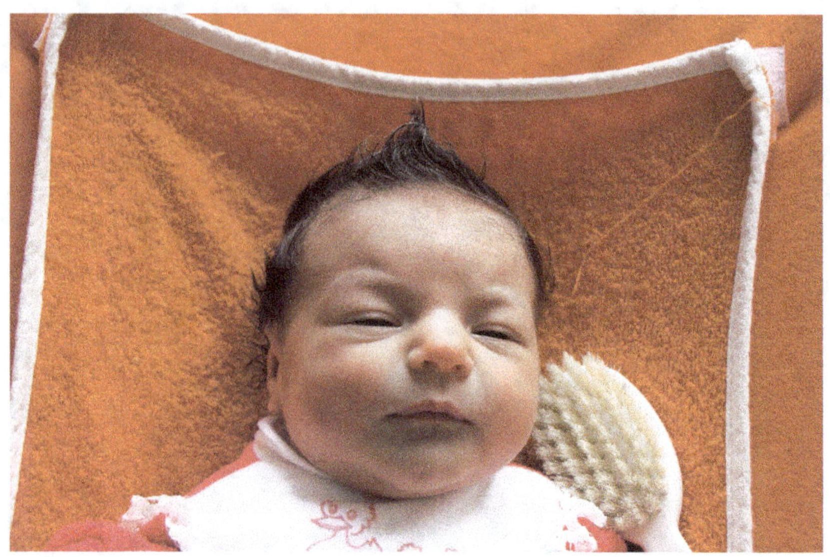

When you go to be tired bed and wake up refreshed the next morning, this only means that you were able to get enough sleep. But when you wake up with a heavy feeling, it only means that you either did not have enough or too much sleep.

A person needs to sleep. Sleeping is the main way of debriefing and resting and it is encouraged. Like all things that are needed, it must also be limited.

Physical activity that a person can perform sometimes is affected by how much time a person was able to sleep. According to studies, sleep can greatly affect a person's ability to function in a day.

A person lacking sleep may not be alert enough to be able to function properly and may commit greater errors as compared to that of a person who had enough sleep the previous night.

The optimal amount of a person's sleeping time can be determined by age as well as how well their circadian rhythm is functioning. Our optimal sleeping time is at its highest while we are young and slowly decreases when we age.

For a newborn baby, a child below one month old, they are in need of12 to 18 hours of sleep on average. They need sleep greater than they need to be awake.

An infant, a child who is still under one year old, is in need of 14 to 15 hours of sleep. Toddlers on the other hand (aged 1-3 years old), are in need of 12 to 14 hours of sleep. Sleep at their age is needed for continuous growth and development.

Pre-schoolers (aged 3-5), are in need of lesser amount of sleep at 11 to 13 hours. When they reach the school age (aged 5-10), they are only in need of 10 to 11 hours of sleep.

For adolescents (aged 10 to 19), the optimal time for sleep is decreased to 8.5 to 9 hours.

Adults need about 7 to 9 hours of sleep per night. This amount of time is also applicable to the elderly. Having an exact amount of sleep every night means that your circadian rhythm is working perfectly.

Your circadian rhythm helps in keeping your brain and body functions in check. It is considered your very own body clock. It makes sure that you are awake on the time that you should be and asleep when you need to rest.

Aside from the correct amount of sleep that a person must get every night, experts also suggest that individuals must make time to take a nap in the middle of the day or right after lunch.

A nap after lunch is greatly advantageous because your brain function decreases after you eat a meal. It is due to the fact that most of your blood pools or is used by your digestive system thus reducing blood and oxygen supply to the brain.

According to studies, taking a nap during the day has been seen to decrease coronary mortality which is possible due to reduced stress to the heart when body functions are decreased when sleeping.

CHAPTER 3- BEAT CHRONIC FATIGUE - SLEEP DEEPER TO WAKE UP BETTER

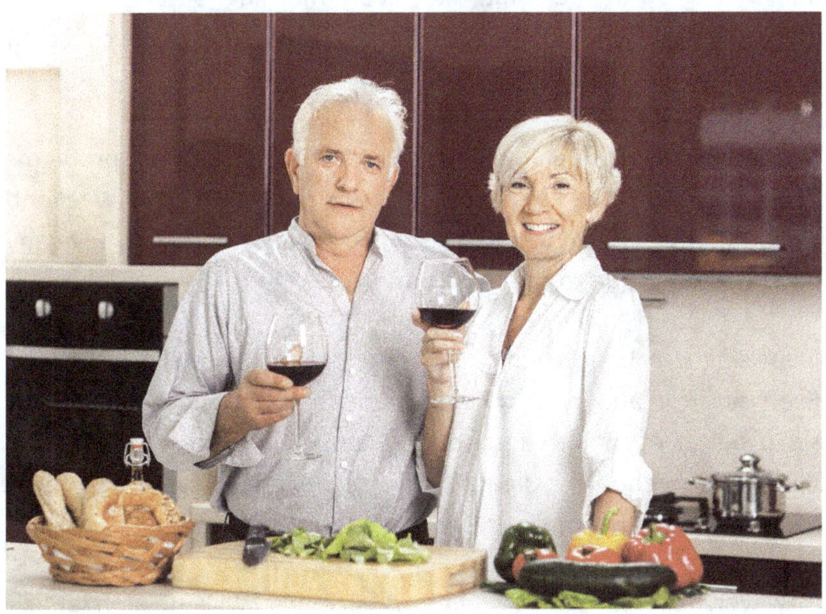

Still tossing around in bed even though you turned in a couple of hours ago? Do you feel uncomfortable and something keeps on bothering you every time you close your eyes? It may be that your circadian rhythm has been disrupted or certain factors have been affecting your sleep time.

There are different ways for a person to be able to sleep comfortably and wake up refreshed the next day. According to the National Sleep Foundation, you have a better chance of sleeping better and deeper when you follow the following:

Schedule, Exercise, Stimulant avoidance, relaxing before sleep, sleeping until sunlight, don't lie in bed, room temperature control, and consultation.

Sleep Better

Setting a schedule means setting your sleeping time every night and waking up at the same time every morning. Setting the time helps your body adapt to the schedule and allows your circadian rhythm to work properly.

Disruption in the sleeping schedule may cause sleeping problems or lead to insomnia. Keeping the schedule up during the weekend will also be beneficial to the person because they will not have any problems adjusting to the new routine on Monday.

Exercising has been seen to affect a person's sleeping schedule. Exercising for about 20 to 30 minutes a day often helps people sleep better at night. Exercise has been seen to help in releasing hormones needed for sleep. It is also beneficial for a person to exercise in the afternoon or 5 to 6 hours before sleeping.

However, exercising right before sleeping will no longer be beneficial for the person involved.

Avoiding caffeine, nicotine, and alcohol to have a good night's sleep all have the same reasons. It affects the individual's sleeping pattern. Caffeine is a substance commonly found in coffee, chocolate, soft drinks, non-herbal teas, diet drugs and some pain relievers. Caffeine stimulates the brain and when the brain is stimulated, it would be hard for the individual to be able to sleep properly.

Smokers tend to sleep lightly and often wake up early in the morning due to nicotine withdrawal. Alcohol robs the individual of deep sleep and REM sleep thus making the person wake up in the middle of the night.

Relaxing before bedtime allows the brain to slip into sleep quicker and allows deeper sleep. A warm bath, relaxing atmosphere, reading and even putting on music make it easier for the person to fall asleep.

Creating a relaxation ritual paired with correct sleeping schedule will definitely allow a good night sleep. Also, sleeping until sunlight can help in the routine. Sunlight or bright lights helps the body's biological clock reset itself every morning.

When you are unable to sleep, lying in bed and doing nothing will not do you any good. Do something else by reading a book, listening to music, watching television until you feel tired helps.

Lying in bed and not doing anything increases a person's anxiety thus reducing the chance for a person to be able to achieve deep sleep. Controlling room temperature provides comfort. If it is too warm or too cold, you would not be able to sleep properly or deeply. Experts suggest that having the right temperature will help you sleep nicely.

When still having trouble sleeping and the previous suggestions are not applicable, it is best to consult your doctor or an expert for that matter. Your physician would be able to help you. Remember, sleep is an important part of your day. To lose it means losing the day ahead.

Chapter 4- Beat Chronic Fatigue – Fight Insomnia

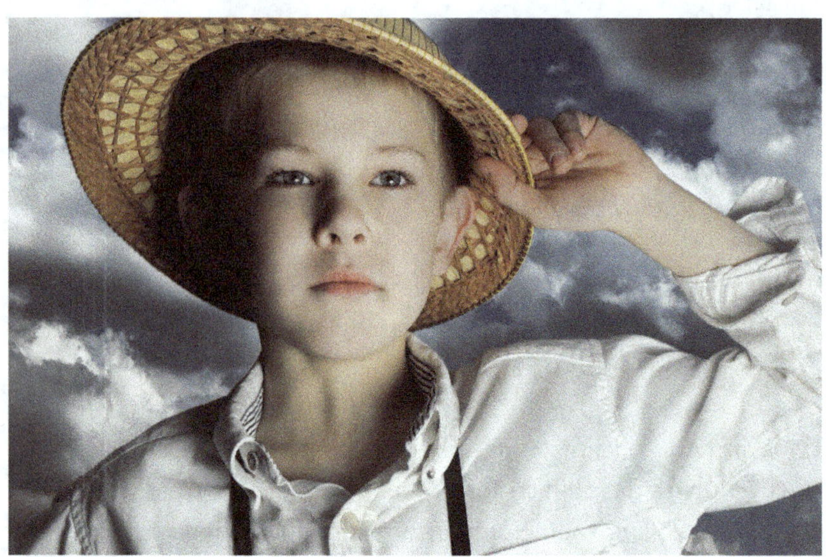

Been tossing and turning in your bed lately? Do you have trouble keeping your eyes shut at night or even falling asleep? Does a little sound outside your window jolt you awake? You might want to check it out because you might be suffering from insomnia.

Insomnia or sleeplessness is a sleeping disorder characterized by a person's inability to fall asleep or stay asleep as long as they want to.

Insomnia may be considered a sign or symptom and may accompany several sleeps, medical and psychiatric disorders.

Insomnia can occur at any age. Insomnia can cause functional impairment to a person who has been experiencing these symptoms.

Insomnia

Insomnia is classified into three groups: transient, acute, and chronic. Transient insomnia has the shortest time. It usually lasts for less than a week and it can be caused by another disorder, changes in sleeping environment, timing of sleep, severe depression or by stress.

An acute insomnia, on the other hand, is the inability to sleep consistently for less than a month. An individual is unable to maintain consistency despite adequate opportunity and circumstances for sleep. This may result in impaired daytime function. Acute insomnia is also called short term insomnia or stress related insomnia. Chronic insomnia is a type of insomnia that lasts for more than a month.

It may be a primary disorder or caused by a medical or psychiatric disorder. Their effects vary according to its cases and severity. Effects may include fatigue and hallucinations.

Among the most common ways of relieving insomnia are Cognitive Behavior Therapy (CBT), Pharmacological and alternative treatment. Cognitive Behavior therapy is a therapy directed towards improved sleeping habits without using pharmacological help. In this therapy, patients are taught ways to improve sleeping habits and relieve counter-productive assumptions about sleep. It allows the person to take control of his sleeping and waking habits, giving them power and making them realize that it is up to them to help themselves.

Pharmacologic treatments include benzodiazepines, non-benzodiazepines, antidepressants, antihistamines such as diphenhydramine, and melatonin to improve sleep.

Each medication prescribed is given according to what the person needs. Combinations of the drugs may be given if it is needed. The use of pharmacological treatments is oftentimes discouraged by physicians due to the possibility of tolerance and dependence of a person to a drug.

Tolerance means the body would need increased dosages of the drug because the initial dose is no longer effective. Dependence is when the individual would resort to medicine use even though it is not needed. Doctors and physicians nowadays create ways to limit the side effects of the drugs by decreasing the dosage when the person is able to sleep on his own.

Alternative treatments make use of herbal treatments in lieu of medications. The use of milk, teas, and other relaxation techniques has been suggested by experts. Milk has a sedative effect which can help an individual fall asleep better. Teas and herbs such as chamomile, valerian, lavender and hops have been introduced to the public and are seen as a better alternative than medications.

Chapter 5- Beat Chronic Fatigue – Be Fit and Healthy

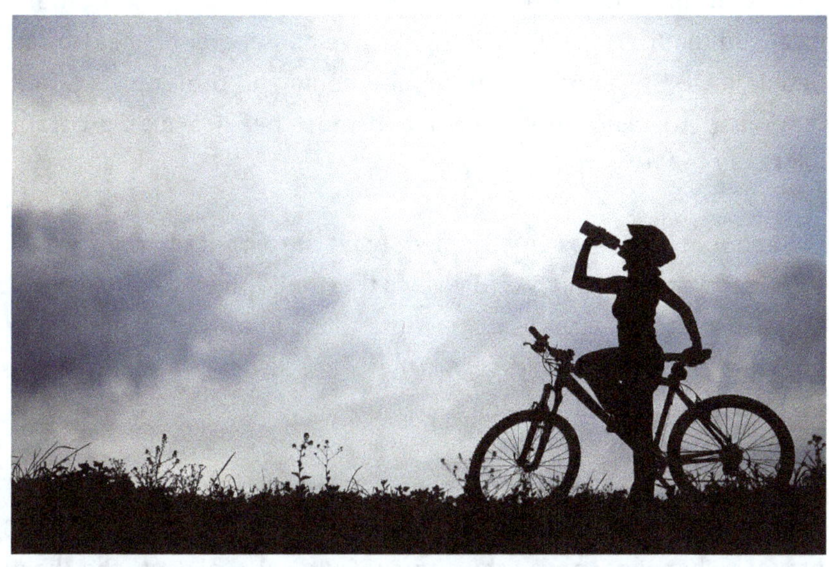

Having a healthy diet is necessary to every human's everyday life. Whatever your reasons are for doing it, you are doing the best thing for yourself. It can be that you aim to lose weight or maybe you plainly want to have a life that is free from any kind of sickness and ailments. Having a daily healthy diet will definitely give you what your little heart's desire.

What most people have is a busy kind of lifestyle and in order to keep up with everything they need the right type of energy providing foods.

What other people may not be aware of is that your energy is boosted with a healthy diet. If your usual diet consists of processed foods or those that are greasy and straight from takeout counters, you are depriving yourself from the nutrients your body needs.

Good Diet

Having a healthy diet allows you to have a body in tip top shape and far from diseases which makes you weak. If you consume a balanced diet daily, you will live an active and energetic life. Not all people have the same dietary requirements and preference. Some may need to lose more weight and must be in a diet program which should be strictly followed.

For some, when diet is mentioned, what automatically registers in their mind are the unflavorful dishes they need to eat which causes them to quit dieting. Although there are dietary programs which may require less salt and sugar, there are also a lot of nutritious foods that can be consumed.

Fresh fruits and vegetables are always the first on the list. As the saying says, "An apple a day keeps the doctor away". Apples, oranges, bananas and other tasty fruits are always the best nutrient providing foods and energy builders too. You just have to continue eating them daily for you to have a fit body.

Healthy food allows your body to function perfectly including your blood flow. Avoiding unhealthy foods means no dangerous cholesterol inside your body as well as the excess fats which slow circulation. With everything that is working as it should, there is no reason for you to be weak and slow moving. You will be full of energy and all charged up because of what you have in you.

Variety is also a good way to keep your body fit. Learning about other foods that provide useful nutrients will allow you to enjoy living a healthy life.

Eating the same kind of fruit everyday will lessen your interest with what you are doing. But if you come up with a variety of dishes that contains nutritious ingredients, you will even love the experience more.

Focusing on what you want will allow you to reach your destination. With a body full of energy, you will be able to fulfill everything that needs to be done. Who would want to live an unhealthy life that is full of worries and sickness?

A healthy body is a healthy mind and when you have a healthy mind mistakes are lessen therefore success should be near.

Chapter 6- Beat Chronic Fatigue – Energized with Exercise

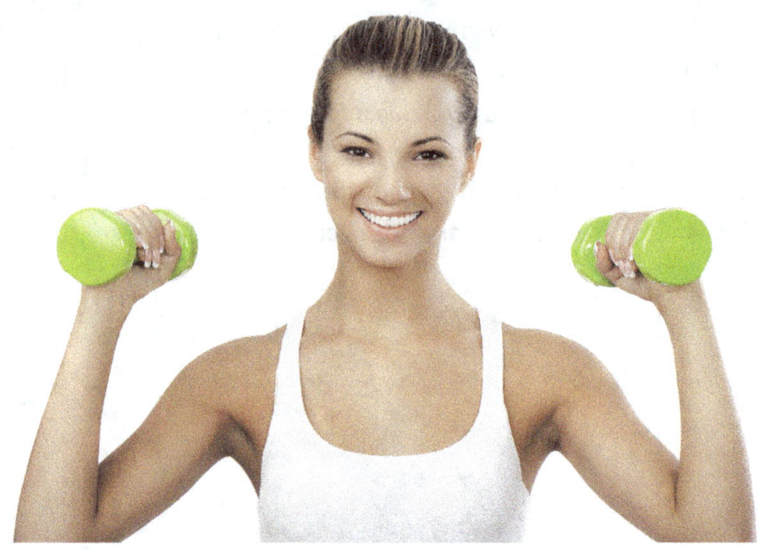

It is a fast paced world that we move in nowadays. No matter how much we try, demands on our time would always become our problem. We no longer have time to have fun, relax or even have a long break that we deserve. These demands may take a toll on both our body and mind. We may later on feel physical or mental fatigue. Experts say that in order to stay fit and healthy in a demanding situation, we must create ways to ensure that we remain fit and mentally sturdy.

Energy

Exercise is a great way to fight stress, reduce fatigue, and increase our everyday energy levels. Even a few minutes spent on stretching those biceps and flexing those hamstrings can certainly help develop that. Studies have shown that there is a direct relationship between exercise and easy fatigability. Physically active people are more likely to have reduced risk for fatigue as compared to physically inactive ones.

Exercise was also seen to have an effect towards the energy level of people with chronic illness like cancer and heart disease. An additional 15 minute walk in their routine is said to increase their capacity to deal with fatigue and stress.

The trick, as experts have said, is exercising when you feel tired. Tired people are less likely to put on their sneakers and go for a run or take the stairs instead of the elevator. Even a little increase in your activities can be helpful.

Little exercises can be included in your routine without wasting much of your time. You can walk to work or ride a bicycle if it is a considerable distance instead of taking your car or taking a cab. You may also climb the stairs rather than take the elevator. Experts say that climbing the stairs for two minutes is equivalent to a 15 minute jog.

Also, making sure that you create a routine for you to follow will also help in the long run. You are able to know how many minutes you have left if you want to really go for an exercise of a different magnitude. Consistency must be maintained so as not to disrupt any major part of your routine.

For people wanting to perform short exercises, a simple run can be continued with a few minutes of stretching, curl ups and pushups.

The whole body must be stretched properly as to prevent any pain or irritation after the exercise. You may also do a couple of pushups and curl ups. You may also perform a couple of weight lifting activities but be careful not to over exert yourself too much. Also, for people wanting exercises that are easy to follow, a few minutes of instructional yoga, kick boxing, aerobics and other instructional exercises may be effective for you.

It is always good to remember to have some time to yourself. And it is always good to spend that free time on taking care of yourself and improving. A few minutes of exercise will always go a long way if you want to be as fit and healthy always.

Chapter 7- Beat Chronic Fatigue – Peaceful Meditation

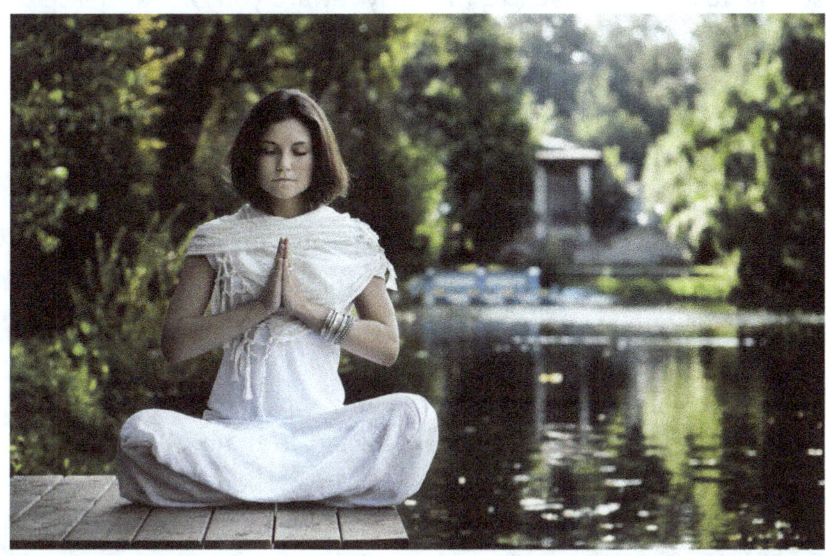

Sometimes with all the issues in life and things to keep up life becomes similar to a roller coaster ride. Having all these in your mind, you tend to stay in bed all night fully awake and having a hard time putting yourself to sleep.

You should never deprive yourself of sleep and a good rest, without having that, you will wake up the next day feeling down, cranky or impatient. This is not something healthy for you, your family and your work.

With so many things on your mind it is impossible for you to relax even during the time you close your eyes. There are people who fix on little things and consider them a life threatening situation if it is undone which causes them to stop relaxing even if there is a need to do so. These are people who even worry about things if their backs are already touching the bed.

Meditation

You need to understand how important sleep is and you must submit yourself on practices that may reward you with a chance to prioritize daily rest and good night's sleep. If your mind always floats back to your issues at work or your family problem even if your body is already telling you to sleep, maybe it is time for you to start meditating.

Pressure is what keeps your mind wandering off instead of getting to rest. Practicing meditation can truly provide you with the solution your body needs.

Taking sleeping pills is not a healthy option since it can be dangerous to you if you become addicted to them. Meditation on the other hand will allow you to have a good sleep.

Practicing meditation before sleep and also after waking up will allow you to have a relaxed mind. It may be a little difficult when you are still starting but as you get used to it, it will work like magic.

It always starts by preparing yourself for your intention. Giving yourself a relaxing bath and making your whole body calm by massaging your arms, hands and all the other parts of your body which you feel stressed and tired.

When you finally feel your entire body is comfortable and nothing feels stiff you can sit down on a chair with your back straight. Let your feet touch the floor firmly and then close your eyes taking long and steady breath in and out of the nose. Repeating this three to five times will help clear what is in your mind.

When you are freeing your mind from all your worries you can breathe in slowly counting to three and then breath it out counting up to six and do this breathing pattern seven more times.

After this, lie on the bed with your stomach touching it with your arms folded and cheeks resting on them. Just focus on the rising and falling of your breathing and allow your mind to dwell on that relaxing moment.

Once you have gotten used to this, you can also try just sitting down while you meditate and relax yourself. Doing this daily before sleep and when you wake up will absolutely free your mind from stressful concern. A healthier happy you will come out from it too.

Chapter 8- Beat Chronic Fatigue – Get Body Clock Working

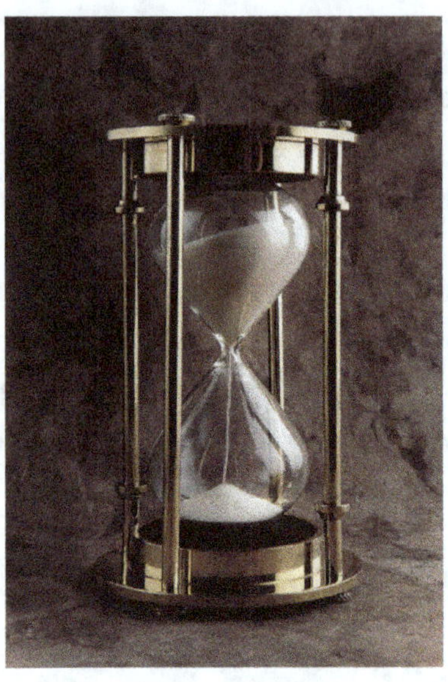

Normally, people rely on alarm clocks if they want to wake up early. It seems that it is impossible to be awake at an early hour without any use of any electronic or those technical devices and gadgets which have alarms.

People are normally dependent on clocks not to be late for meetings, school and work but they should know that there is a better way to set an alarm on a particular hour without the use of any kind of watches or clocks.

The word "biological clock" may be something you have heard of before. This is the internal clock of human beings which tells the body to sleep when it is time to sleep or get up if it's time to wake up.

The same with animals, they also have biological clocks which they follow every day making them wake up exactly the same time every day. The problem with our biological clock though is it has a lot of barriers making it "not work" the same way as how it works on animals.

Biological Clock

These are still our capabilities and abilities that hinders it to work properly overriding its ticking. But with serious focus and practice, we can use our own mind to set our mental clock. This may sound uncommon but it can be done. For sure you have met someone who wakes up the same time every day unless he is sick and needs to stay in bed to rest.

That is exactly what will come out of you if you program your mind to think that way. Just channel your mind into something you want done and it will naturally cooperate. Of course there are some preparations that need to be considered if you want to succeed and be able to have an operational mental alarm in you.

If you want to be able to do it, you may follow these steps.

1. First, you need to be in bed early free of noise and interruption. Your main intention here is to relax yourself and give it a good rest your mind to focus on your intention.

2. Set your mind and body in a relaxing mode. It would be easier if you start from one part to the other starting from the top. This method is also known as "entering the alpha level". You need to breathe deeply and start making your whole body relax. You will know if you are able to reach that state since your mind will not be occupied with anything else. It takes practice though but doing this daily will make this process a lot easier as well as faster.

3. Think of somewhere you would like to be when you want to relax. That will allow you to keep yourself calm and relax.

4. Picture a clock set in a particular time you want to wake up. It can be any kind of clock or watch as long as it is the one that you fancy.

5. Command yourself to wake up at that particular hour you set your mental clock to and you will wake up the next day on that very hour.

Chapter 9- Beat Chronic Fatigue: Manage Stress

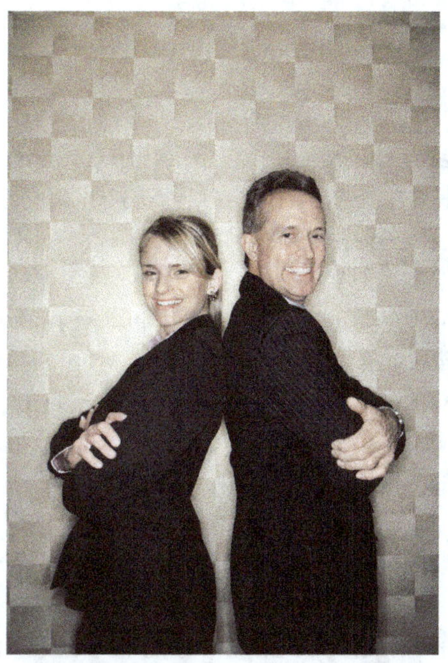

Have you ever seen a successful corporate executive who does not look slick and stress free? Rarely can you tell when they are stressed out and that is because they expertly learned how to successfully manage the level of stress they are in.

They are smart enough to know that if they walk around in a disarrayed state and let their subordinates see them that way, these people will also be affected or doubt their leadership capabilities too.

You do not need to be a corporate executive to be able to battle stress and appear great in front of people. You can actually find a way to eliminate your worries and stress producing concerns and live a happy life each and every day.

How To Beat Chronic Fatigue

You must first understand that there are two types of stress and be able to identify which is which. Eustress also known as positive stress is the type of stress we need for our health. The one we need to stop doing is called episodic acute stress.

Being Smarter

Stress in general is the reaction of the body by releasing a sudden energy burst which causes hormones to shuffle and this can be draining if it becomes too much.

Eustress is giving you a positive effect since it makes you relax and allows you to feel positive such as bungee jumping, going out on your first date with a long time crush or just simply having a quick speedy slide down the ski slope. Anything that can make you feels the rush and makes your adrenaline pump.

Episodic acute stress on the other hand is the type that drains your energy with no positivity in it. Dwelling on an unfortunate event of your life or worrying about unpaid bills is one of them. If you are smart enough how to turn all these negatively causing issues into something that will become beneficial to you, you will be free from the stress that eats you up causing you to become unproductive.

Once you realize how to determine the type of stress you are in, you can easily find ways to remove or at least minimize the effects it will do for you.

But in order for you to do that, you need to have a healthy mind to come up with working ideas. Living a healthy life is the key to this. Eating the right kind of food and doing exercise will allow you to live in this state of health.

Remember that the reason why you are in a stressful situation is because you were not able to foresee the events that caused it. If your mind is clear from worries and useless concerns, you will have a backup plan to solve it in case it arises. The smart way to deal with stress is absolutely having a relaxed healthy life.

There will be times that you will be affected by it because that is normal, but being resilient is something that you can be. A healthy mind will give you ideas to bounce back and get back on the race again.

CHAPTER 10- PAIN AND CHRONIC FATIGUE

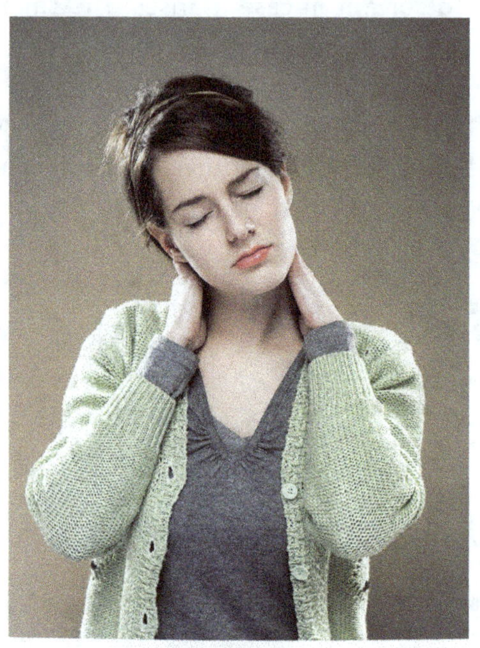

The word pain can be used in many different ways, so it is probably worth defining exactly we mean by the word pain in the context of this report.

Throughout this report, I am dealing with physical pain as opposed to the kind of general life-encompassing suffering that can make every day a misery. The type of pain we are talking about here does not for example include the kind of pain that you might suffer if you have no money or are homeless, emotional desperation brought on by family bereavement and so on

As we have all felt physical pain from time to time, we all know what it is but finding an accurate definition is actually far harder than it might at first appear like it should be.

For example, whilst the International Association for the Study of Pain defines it as 'an unpleasant sensory and emotional experience associated with actual or potential tissue damage, or described in terms of such damage', it is important to understand that pain is actually highly subjective.

What one person might consider an agonizing pain could be nothing more than a minor irritant to someone else, and people who suffer from chronic pain every day gradually forget about it to some degree even though the pain does not go away.

For this reason, it is sometimes suggested that the definition provided by a noted pain control expert Margo McCaffrey in 1968 might be viewed as more accurate. She said that 'pain is whatever the experiencing person says it is, existing whenever he says it does'.

What is certainly indisputable is the fact that almost half of visits to doctors and medical practitioners in the USA every year are as a result of a pain problem that the patient wants solving.

When this happens, your doctor will usually do two things.

Firstly, they will try to characterize the pain itself using various different criteria or descriptions such as intensity, type of pain (throbbing, dull, burning etc), reason for the pain and bodily location.

After asking these questions, if there is no clear reason for the pain, they will examine you to find out why you are suffering the way you are as there is clearly some underlying reason for your pain of which you are not fully aware.

How To Beat Chronic Fatigue

Generally speaking, pain will go away with simple treatments such as rest and of course through the use of painkilling analgesic medicines. However, we have already seen that many people suffer chronic pain, a pain that becomes a medical condition in itself and does not go away of its own accord or as a result of simple treatments.

Pain is an essential part of the body's defense mechanism, a natural reflex reaction telling you to back off from something that has the potential to cause damage to you. Furthermore, it also help you to change your behavior so that whatever it was that caused you pain is not repeated, thereby protecting against further physical harm or damage.

Pain is a conscious sensation – sometimes we are too conscious of it, and it can strike anytime, anywhere, either as a result of a traumatic accident or because of the sudden or gradual onset of an unexpected medical problem.

Perhaps surprisingly, it is generally believed that when we are born, every human being already has built-in natural pain control mechanisms.

Furthermore, it is posited that in our caveman days, these natural pain management processes or substances (hormones, enzymes and other naturally occurring chemicals in the body) would be activated almost from birth because the need to protect themselves against harm and pain was so much greater in those days.

After all, even then, millions of years ago, our antecedents felt pain but they did not have aspirin or ibuprofen that they could take to get rid of it when pain struck. Whilst some suggest that herbal remedies for pain relief date from these times, it is still nevertheless the fact that people back then had far less in the way of effective pain relief available, hence the belief that natural pain control mechanisms were far more prevalent.

This is important to understand because more recent research has built on this by indicating that these natural mechanisms have not entirely disappeared.

However, the world that a newborn baby arrives in is nowadays a very different world to that of our caveman forbears. Thus, there is some evidence that modern life simply fails to 'switch on' these natural pain control processes.

This was highlighted in a study at the University of Maryland in Baltimore which indicated that sugar and suckling activate these natural pain control processes in very young babies. Furthermore, they also established that these control mechanisms seem to have something to do with the spinal column, although as the research was not conducted on human beings, the exact relevance of this to man has still to be established with any degree of certainty.

Nevertheless, the research suggested that a few minutes of suckling and the rendition of sugar water to babies could significantly reduce the level of pain felt by laboratory animals a few moments later.

This is an important consideration for any expectant parents as it suggests that from the day that baby is born, it is possible to build up their natural resistance to pain relatively quickly and easily.

Whilst there clearly needs to be more study on this, it is definitely something to bear in mind if you are an expert parent or anticipate becoming one.

CHAPTER 11- PAINKILLER: CHRONIC FATIGUE SOLUTION?

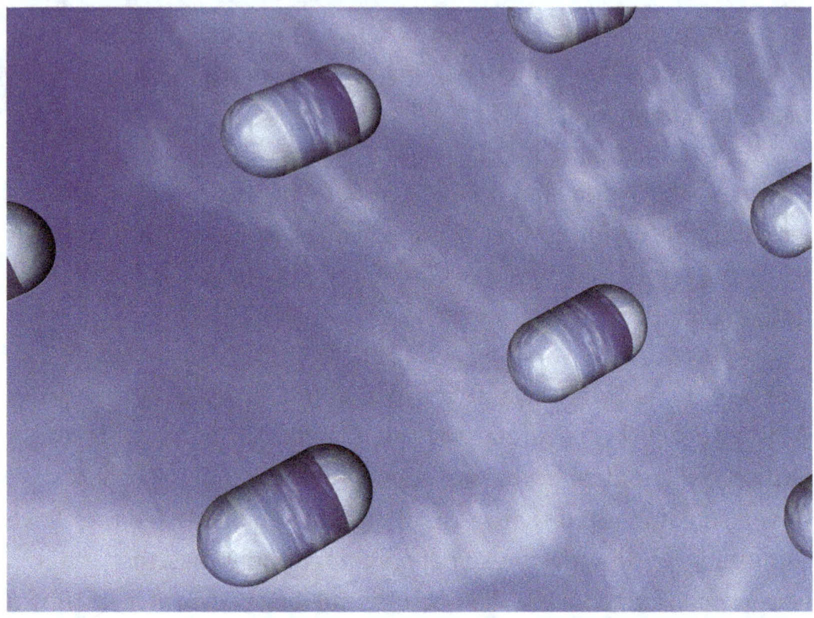

Aspirin is still one of the most widely used analgesic painkillers and as you can buy aspirin in almost any convenience store; it is a medicine that thousands of people all over the world use whenever they have a minor pain such as a headache or some other similar condition.

Technically speaking, aspirin is a non-steroidal anti-inflammatory drug (an NSAID) and was the first drug of its type to be discovered and isolated. For the vast majority of people, aspirin is a relatively safe medicine to take, although as previously suggested, it is a medicine to be avoided for people who are already taking other medicines with which it might interact.

In addition however, it is estimated that approximately 1% of people suffer from an aspirin allergy which is most commonly seen on the skin in the form of hives, rashes, and swellings. An aspirin allergy can bring on asthma attacks in people who already have a susceptibility to asthma, with an estimated 10% of asthma sufferers likely to suffer this form of allergic reaction to aspirin. This can extend as far as developing into anaphylaxis (a severe life-threatening allergic reaction) in a worst- case scenario.

Aspirin can also cause upset stomachs and diarrhea, as well as bleeding (both internal and external) and bruising as a result of its anticoagulant capabilities.

In a very small number of cases, aspirin can lead to Reyes' Syndrome which is a potentially fatal condition characterized by damage to many internal organs, especially the liver and the brain. Given the seriousness of this particular condition, early diagnosis of Reye's Syndrome is absolutely essential because otherwise brain damage or death could be the result.

Reye's syndrome passes through five distinct stages with the first being characterized by heavy vomiting that is not reversed by eating, general lethargy, nightmares and all-round confusion. If anyone who is taking aspirin exhibits any of these symptoms, it is absolutely critical to get them to a doctor or emergency hospital as quickly as possible.

Paracetomol (and Tylenol) (acetaminophen) is another widely used and generally available analgesic as well as being effective for reducing fever as well. For this reason, it is widely used as a treatment for headaches, fever and other minor aches and pains.

Paracetamol is technically known as an aniline analgesic and is the only one still widely used for the treatment of pain, because all other similar analgesics were withdrawn as they were believed to exhibit carcinogenic qualities (which so far, paracetamol does not). However, the fact that it is made from coal tar may give you a reason to question this as carbon is often believed to have carcinogenic qualities as well.

In normal doses, one of the advantages of paracetamol is that it does not irritate the stomach lining or affect blood coagulation in the same way that NSAID's like aspirin do.

However, higher than recommended usage has been seen to have a potential connection with gastrointestinal bleeding and very high dosages have the capacity to cause liver damage, which in the most severe cases can be fatal. Indeed, paracetamol or Tylenol poisoning is the number one cause of acute liver failure in most Western countries and the way that most people choose to commit suicide in these countries as well.

Furthermore, a massive study conducted in 31 countries and involving over 200,000 children in 2008 and reported in the leading medical journal 'The Lance t ' found that the use of paracetamol in the first year of life made children far more likely to develop asthmatic symptoms at around age six or seven. In addition, children who took paracetamol during the first year of life and also children who took the drug at ages 6-7 demonstrated a far higher likelihood of developing eczema and rhino conjunctivitis later too.

Ibuprofen (Advil, Nuprin etc) and Naproxen (Aleve) are both NSAID's like aspirin. They therefore share many of the potential side effects that have already been highlighted as been endemic to aspirin. For instance, aspirin allergy, upset stomach and a higher risk of asthma attacks can be equally ascribed to both of these medicines as they can to aspirin.

Ibuprofen however carries additional risks as it is believed to increase the risk of myocardial infarction (heart attack) if taken in high dosages and you can also cause or exacerbate irritable bowel syndrome, Crohn's disease and ulcerative colitis due to its capability of starting gastrointestinal bleeding.

With Naproxen, some of the most widely reported side-effects include constipation or diarrhea, drowsiness, upset stomach, stuffy nose and heartburn.

However, whilst the NSAID's already detailed are likely to carry a slight increase in risk levels for heart attacks and strokes, the risk associated with Naproxen might be considerably more serious. Indeed, the National Institute of Health terminated a trial into the effects of Naproxen as a drug for reducing the severity of Alzheimer's disease (in 2006) because of the suspicion that the drug significantly increased the risk of heart attack or stroke.

Since that time, further analysis suggests that at normal dosages, the increased risk of suffering a heart attack or stroke is fairly low although as you will see in the next section, this is certainly not true of all NSAID's.

Prescription drugs

As a general observation, most of the pharmaceutical painkillers that are prescribed by doctors fall into one of two categories.

The first group is made up of stronger non-steroidal anti-inflammatory drugs than those that are available across the counter such as aspirin and ibuprofen. The second group of drugs that your doctor may prescribe to deal with your pain is the opiate or synthetic opiate-based drugs.

Let's take each in turn starting with a small selection of the more common NSAID's that your doctor might prescribe.

Celecoxib (Celebrex), Diclofenac (Volteran, Naklofen, Arbitren etc) and Tramadol (Ultram) are all NSAID's that bring with them the usual potential adverse side-effects of taking drugs of this nature such as an increased risk of internal and external bleeding, bruising, upset stomachs, constipation and nausea etc.

However, unlike Naproxen with which it now appears that the increased risk of suffering a heart attack or stroke at normal dosage is small, the risk is significantly higher with both Celecoxib and Diclofenac.

Furthermore, the risk seems to be increased irrespective of the dosage although of course the risk is going to become larger as your dosage is increased.

Research indicates that the increased heart attack and stroke risk factor is 1.63 compared to non-users. Nevertheless, this represents an increased risk that it is suggested many chronic pain sufferers will tolerate in return for the greater pain management capabilities of these drugs in comparison to weaker drugs such as aspirin. In effect, it seems that many pain sufferers know the increased risks and are willing to live with them to get rid of their pain.

In addition, the risk of suffering liver or kidney damage appears to be increased with all three drugs included in this category and should such damage occur, it appears that in most cases, it is likely to be irreversible.

Demerol, Vicodin and Lorcet are all drugs that are based on natural or synthetic opiate based drugs that are used to treat various different medical conditions and pain caused by these conditions.

Demerol is a drug that contains pethidine which for the majority of the 20th century was the most commonly favored opiate based drug, with 60% of doctors being reported as prescribing it for acute pain and 23% prescribing it for chronic pain in 1983. The popularity of the drug stemmed from the fact that it was supposed to be safer whilst also being stronger than morphine-based drugs which were the major alternative available at the time.

Since that time however, this has been proved incorrect. Indeed, because of the short duration of its effectiveness and low potency, it is debatable whether Demerol was ever really effective at all.

On the other hand, it carries a far more significant risk of causing neuropath logical problems such as delirium and seizures than many other competing medicines; hence it is only prescribed very rarely nowadays. In fact, several countries such as Australia have either placed severe limits on the use of Demerol or banned it altogether.

The side effects of Vicodin are fortunately not as severe as those of Demerol, with the most common being nausea, upset stomach, light- headedness or dizziness. In more rare cases, Vicodin can cause allergic reactions, unconsciousness, jaundice, bleeding, bruising, constipation and altered sex drive, but these are the exceptions, rather than the norm.

One Vicodin problem that is significant is the fact that it is a drug to which it is easy to develop resistance relatively quickly. Consequently, many people are tempted to take progressively larger doses of Vicodin in an effort to combat the effects of increasing bodily familiarity with the drug which will naturally decrease its effectiveness.

Whilst increasing the dosage in this way will fight the pain more quickly and more effectively, all opiate-based drugs are addictive and obviously, the more of them you take, the more quickly it is likely that you become addicted. Vicodin can be highly addictive due to the presence of hydrocodone but whilst increasing the rate at which you take the drug to alleviate your pain will work, the damaging effects in both social and medical terms could be extremely harmful.

Becoming addicted to Vicodin represents a classic case of being addicted to prescription drugs and even though this is a prescribed drug, this does not make the addiction any worse. For example, reports of significant social and legal problems for Vicodin addiction sufferers are common as they visit doctor after doctor after doctor to try to get a prescription to feed their increasingly ravenous appetite

The 'potential adverse side-effects' of Vicodin therefore go way beyond the short term physical or medical side-effects highlighted earlier.

Rather, they encompass many far more damaging side-effects which can and will adversely affect the quality of your life if you become addicted to this particular drug.

Remember, all opiate based drugs are naturally addictive so you must always apply a great deal of caution with any drug of this type.

As suggested, the ingredient in Vicodin that makes it so addictive is hydrocodone, and if you followed the earlier link, you may have noticed that amongst the brand names that are associated with this particular drug is Lorcet.

Hence, this particular medicine also has significant addictive qualities too. Addicts often demonstrate serious liver problems whilst an overdose of Lorcet or any other hydrocodone-based medicine can lead to respiratory depression, heart failure, heart attack, jaundice, seizures, blackouts, amnesia and ultimately death.

Furthermore, because many opiate-based drugs include acetaminophen (our old friend paracetamol or Tylenol), even relatively minor over- doses have the capability of causing jaundice or even serious, irreversible liver damage in many patients.

To sum up…

All pharmaceutical analgesics have potential side-effects, ranging from relatively mild problems such as upset stomachs or a touch of diarrhea to serious, irreversible problems like liver or heart failure, drug addiction and death.

Of course, for the vast majority of people, most of the worst side-effects of taking chemical-based pharmaceutical analgesics are never likely to be something that affects them. Nevertheless, the fact is, if only one in a hundred people suffers an allergic reaction to aspirin or one in 10 finds that their asthma has been exacerbated by taking the same drug, the odds of suffering an adverse side-effect are probably far higher than you had ever previously imagined.

The case for avoiding these drugs if at all possible is therefore extremely strong which brings us to the point of considering what alternatives there might be. Fortunately, there are many entirely natural alternatives available for anyone who is looking for effective pain management and these alternatives will provide the focus for the rest of this book.

CHAPTER 12- HOW TO BETTER MANAGE PAIN TO PREVENT FATIGUE

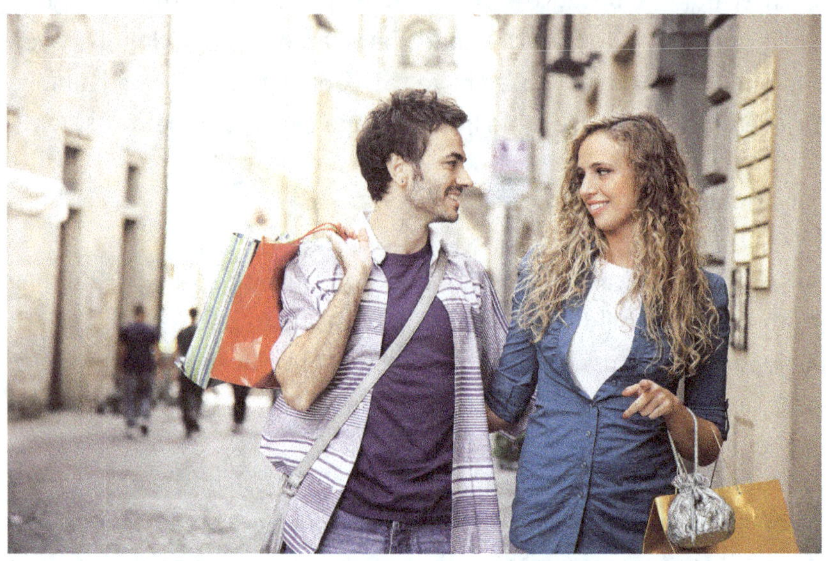

One important consideration that your doctor will take into account before they prescribe pharmaceutical analgesics is the type of pain that you are suffering from.

They will take into account whether it is a chronic or acute pain and whether there is any underlying condition or situation that is causing the pain before deciding upon what medicine to give you. A similar situation will apply if you are buying over-the-counter painkillers well, because whilst paracetamol or Tylenol might be very effective for dealing with fever and the pain from and associated with a headache, aspirin will be far less effective for dealing with a fever problem.

Similar considerations apply when you are looking at natural pain management solutions as well because some solutions will work better in some pain management situations than they will in others.

Furthermore, if you have a specific medical condition or situation that is causing pain, some natural pain management solutions are likely to be more appropriate than others.

As an example, the painkilling approach that you use to get rid of a headache or backache is likely to be significantly different to the approach that you adopt if you are trying to combat the pain caused by cancer or it's treatment or the various aches and pains associated with pregnancy and childbirth.

Hence, many of the solutions that are going to be explained are likely to be more effective in certain circumstances or situations than in others.

You need to know what kind of pain it is that you need to combat before deciding upon the best way of using completely natural pain management strategies, tactics and ideas to minimize the adverse effects of your problems.

Massage for pain relief

There are apparently over 80 different styles of massage and body therapy, many of which have been developed by individual practitioners who have taken the original massage idea and developed it as a result of their practical experiences.

Furthermore, there are many associated practices like reflexology and shiatsu which are broadly associated but not entirely synonymous with massage that some people sometimes confuse with massage.

The basic concept of massage as a pain relief strategy is that rubbing and massaging various different points of your body confuses or 'side- tracks' your ability to register pain according to what is known as the 'gate control theory'.

This theory is based upon the concept that pain impulses travel from various different parts of your body through the central nervous system and your spinal column to the brain. It is only when these pain signals arrive in your brain that you register pain although of course, it is a matter of a very small number of nanoseconds between the stimuli happening at some place or point on your body and your brain registering pain.

The 'gate control theory' explanation of why massage works as a pain relief strategy is based on the idea that your body only has the ability to send a certain number of signals to your brain at any one time, and if certain signals do not reach your brain, they will not be 'registered'.

Consequently, when you are enjoying a relaxing massage, the rubbing and stroking sends other far more pleasurable signals to your brain, thus 'populating' the nerves that carry these signals with a positive message leaving no room for the negative pain message to get through.

There is also some evidence that pleasurable massage results in the release of endorphins which are enzymes produced by the pituitary gland, the positive effects of which resemble the effects of opiate drugs. However, as endorphins are entirely natural and their production is strictly controlled by your body, there is no potential harm involved in experiencing the happiness or exhilaration that is often known as an 'endorphin rush'.

Furthermore, endorphins also prevent nerve cells releasing more pain signals, which is for example one of the reasons why top sports people can often continue to compete even when they are injured, because extreme activity allied to excitement prompts the 'rush' that masks the pain.

The following are the forms of massage that are most commonly associated with providing pain relief.

Swedish massage

Swedish massage is a massage style that was first developed in Scandinavia nearly 200 years ago by Pehr Henrik Ling who learned many of the basics that he would later develop into Swedish massage from a Chinese fellow named Ming with whom he sailed for four years.

After returning to Copenhagen, he developed these ideas still further into something similar to what we recognize as Swedish massage which was first brought to the USA in the 1850s.

From just a small handful of Swedish massage clinics in Boston and Washington, they can now be found in almost every city and town throughout the USA (and throughout most other western countries as well). Hence, Swedish massage is the most popular form of massage in the USA and if using this type of massage to bring pain relief sounds like something you might work for you, it should be relatively easy to find a local practitioner.

The basic concept of Swedish massage is that it focuses on long, gliding strokes of the masseuse hands across your skin, with some 'kneading' (the exact same action as if you were making bread) allied to the application of friction techniques to some of the most obvious muscle groups.

Most commonly, the majority of strokes go towards the heart, following the blood flow because there is an emphasis on stimulating blood flow through the soft bodily tissues. This form of massage can be practiced in a relatively vigorous and not so gentle manner or it can be very soft and gentle on the other hand, depending upon circumstances and requirements.

Swedish massage is commonly used to prompt a wide range of benefits including all of the following:

• It helps relax muscles. Hence, if you have a muscle pain caused by stress, tension or even a slight muscle damage, massage can loosen the muscle and thereby reduce the pain and sometimes also the swelling too.

• It can help to reduce the pain from other bodily damage such as fractures, sprains, sciatica, stiff joints and strains. This applies equally to people who have suffered injuries and to those who are simply feeling the adverse effects of getting older!

• There are certain substances in the body that naturally slow down the process of recovering from muscle strains, sprains and damage. Because Swedish massage is effective for removing uric and lactic acid (and other waste products) from your muscles, it helps to speed up the recovery process, meaning that any pain you are suffering will disappear more quickly.

• As Swedish massage can be used to help to stretch muscles, tendons and ligaments, it helps to prevent the kind of damage that might cause pain at a later date. In effect, Swedish massage is not only curative but preventative too.

• In general terms, Swedish massage helps to stimulate improved blood circulation, relaxes the nerves and stimulates the nervous system at one and the same time. It also helps to reduce stress and tension which can be a cause of physical pain as tensed up muscles are far more likely to suffer damage or injury the muscles that are loose and flexible.

The bottom line is that 95% people who undergo Swedish massage leave their session feeling markedly better in many, many different ways, both physically and psychologically.

The benefits of Swedish massage for anyone who is suffering any of the particular types of pain highlighted in the previous list are undeniable. If therefore you are suffering muscle, joint or sprain pains, trying Swedish massage before resorting to analgesic painkillers has got to make sense.

Deep muscle massage

As the name would probably suggest, the concept of deep muscle massage is to work the muscles more thoroughly than is common in Swedish massage, with the ultimate objective being the release of deep muscle tension to reduce potential muscle pain and stress.

Using this particular form of massage, the masseuse will usually use direct pressure or friction allied with slow strokes as a way of 'digging' deeper into the muscles fibers and tissues to alleviate the deepest tension. This is not to suggest that deep muscle massage needs to be painful but it is far more noticeable than Swedish massage, as are the beneficial effects.

With this particular technique, the movements are most commonly carried out across the muscle fibers in a 'cross grain' pattern and applied with the fingers, thumbs or perhaps sometimes even elbows. Because of this, the effects are likely to most beneficial to those who have deep muscle tensions, strains and ache that cause them discomfort or pain. Consequently, if Swedish massage does not really provide the pain relief that you need, it might benefit you to consider going one stage further with deep muscle massage.

Thai massage

Thai massage was originally believed to have originated in India where it was heavily influenced by Ayurvedic ideas and philosophy before migrating to Thailand some 2500 years ago.

From that time to this, the original massage techniques that came from India have been increasingly influenced by traditional Chinese medicine so that what we now recognize as Thai massage represents a physical manifestation of a combination of the two great medical traditions of the East.

With the original antecedents of Thai massage coming from India, you may not find it a great surprise to realize that this particular form of massage is often called Thai Yoga Massage, as some people describe it as undertaking a yoga session without doing the exercise yourself.

It is a form of massage that is considerably more demanding and energizing than Swedish massage for example, which of course means that if you suffer serious physical problems of any form, you should consult your doctor before considering undertaking a Thai massage session.

The massage itself is usually performed whilst the 'patient' is on the floor and involves the masseuse using their hands, legs, knees and feet to provide the massage. In a similar (but different way) to deep muscle massage, Thai massage gets down to the deepest levels of your muscles and joints, providing relief that Swedish massage may not be capable of providing.

People who have undergone Thai massage will tell you that it is both incredibly relaxing and energizing at exactly the same time, and that muscle aches, pains and strains will go away after the initial 'buzz' has subsided.

Once again, if you have muscle pains or aches and Swedish massage does not do the job for you, this is another alternative to consider trying.

Acupuncture – the great pain reliever...

Acupuncture is an ancient Chinese art that had been practiced for thousands of years, one that has been proven on many occasions to be extremely effective for promoting general good health but also for relieving pain of many different types and descriptions.

The first thing to understand about acupuncture is that it is adopts a holistic view of any medical or even psychological problems that you might be suffering, including physical pain.

In essence, whereas a Western doctor will treat the symptoms of that pain by prescribing a drug that attacks only the area where the pain is felt, an acupuncturist adopts the view that the 'something' that has caused your pain is not necessarily located in that particular part of the body. Consequently, they will try to find the root cause of that pain wherever that may be located in your body before dealing with it.

Acupuncture is based on the concept that every human being contains a 'vital energy' flow that courses around their body and that pains, illnesses or sicknesses are signs that this vital energy flow has been disturbed in some way. Vital energy flows along meridians or 'channels' that are recognized by acupuncture to connect certain apparently unconnected parts of the body to one another.

Hence, when a problem that represents a disturbance in the vital energy flow appears, it is logical that the acupuncturist will address that problem by attempting open up the appropriate energy meridian so that the flow can be stimulated and the problem solved.

There are certain points along each of these channels or meridians that are recognized by traditional Chinese acupuncturists as being 'acupupoints', the places where interruptions most commonly occur.

Hence you have the idea that the traditional acupuncturist will insert very fine, long needles through the skin to stimulate these 'acupoints' to free up the vital energy flow.

Nowadays, many traditional acupuncturist still continue with the practice of using needles but there are many alternative forms of acupuncture, such as using small, highly targeted electrical charges on the same 'acupoints' as a way of stimulating the energy flow. Other practitioners have been known to use magnets whilst there is ongoing study and development of using lasers for the same purposes.

One of the problems with acupuncture is that whilst it has been used for in excess of 2000 years as a treatment for pain and illness, it is still not fully understood why acupuncture works as well as it does. Although even medical doctors accept that acupuncture can be a very highly effective treatment for dealing with pain, we (and they) still don't really understand why this should be.

However, as reported in this article, two research studies carried out in the mid-90s provided a very clear indication that for whatever reason acupuncture seems to work so well, it does. This is why the same article reported that acupuncture is the favored nonmedical treatment alternative of the majority of medical doctors.

There are many theories put forward as to why acupuncture can be such an effective treatment for pain in apparently unconnected areas of the body. One of these theories suggests that acupuncture points stimulate the central nervous system which then releases chemicals and hormones into the spinal column and muscles.

It is further posited that these chemicals and hormones alter the experience or perception of pain whilst also stimulating the body's ability to heal itself considerably more quickly than would happen without acupuncture. Hence, the pain relief is more immediate and as the underlying condition is dealt with more quickly, the pain recedes far more swiftly too.

An alternative theory propounded by Western scientists is that there is some evidence that acupuncture points represent the bodies electromagnetic 'junctions'. Hence, by stimulating the junctions, it frees up the flow of electromagnetic charges throughout the body, which in turn appears to stimulate the flow of natural painkilling chemicals such as endorphins.

Other studies have shown that acupuncture appears to alter the chemistry of the brain by prompting the release of neurotransmitters and neuro-hormones. In addition, because it also appears as if acupuncture stimulates subtle changes in your central nervous system's ability to deal with pain, there does seem to be some evidence for why acupuncture seems to be such an effective treatment for pain.

One of the beauties of acupuncture as a natural pain treatment is that unlike massage (as an example), it can be used to treat pain of any type and in any area of the body due to the fact that it is an entirely holistic (whole body) approach to pain management. Whereas as a method of pain relief, massage is very firmly focused on getting rid of muscle pain, acupuncture can be used to address any kind of pain, anywhere in your body.

This is one of the reasons why acupuncture is becoming increasingly widely accepted by the 'traditional' Western medical fraternity who are nowadays increasingly likely to recommend a combination of analgesic painkillers and acupuncture in many situations where pain needs to be dealt with.

For example, this approach is becoming increasingly common for people who suffer post-operative pain. By providing a combination of analgesic painkillers and acupuncture, many doctors have found that they are able to completely rid post-operative patients of pain in a way that analgesics on their own have never been capable of doing at safe   dosage levels.

Unlike many natural techniques for bringing relief from pain, acupuncture can be used to deal with almost any kind of pain, a fact which is often unreported or ignored.

For example, many women report that acupuncture can be highly effective for inducing labor and that many of the pains and stresses of suffering through pregnancy can also be significantly relieved by acupuncture.

Some women suffer back pains or sciatica whilst pregnant because of the additional weight being carried which acupuncture can significantly reduce. Many women also suffer morning sickness and whilst acupuncture will not necessarily get rid of it, it can provide significant help in reducing the nausea levels that most women feel at this time.

It will do this by putting pressure on the Pericardium 6 acupuncture point which is inside the wrist. A strategy that has been proven time and again to reduce all forms of nausea, including that associated with morning sickness.

Incidentally, as an alternative to acupuncture, you might want to consider using a commercially produced acupressure band to put pressure on the same acupuncture point as a way of reducing the nausea of morning sickness.

In the last trimester, many women suffer pelvic girdle pain and according to Swedish studies, acupuncture can help relive these pains too.

The beauty of using acupuncture to reduce the severity of the various aches and pains associated with pregnancy is that by doing so, you reduce or remove the necessity to taking drugs. For some women who are drug intolerant, this is a necessity but even if you do not fall into this category, it obviously makes sense to reduce your reliance on drugs whilst you're carrying baby and during the birth process.

Another area of pain relief that can be dealt with highly effectively and efficiently with acupuncture is the relief of pain for cancer patients.

Because cancer is not one disease (there are over 300 different malignant cancers) and also because chemotherapy treats all of the different forms of cancer in a different way, it is not possible to say that acupuncture is going to be helpful in every case.

Nevertheless, in terms of helping cancer patients get over their pain or the dreaded nausea that is a very common side effect of undergoing chemotherapy, acupuncture can once again be an invaluable additional 'tool' in the pain management toolbox.

As this article concludes by answering the question which it attributes to many cancer patients 'Can acupuncture help me?' it is likely that acupuncture can 'in all probability help in the care of the cancer patient'.

Whilst it is fair to suggest that we still don't really understand why acupuncture is so effective as a treatment for pain, the overwhelming evidence collected over thousands of years from medical experts all over the world is that acupuncture represent a superbly effective way of dealing with pain, almost irrespective of why or how that pain occurs.

If therefore you suffer pain – especially chronic pain that is unlikely to be dealt with by something that provides more temporary relief such as massage – acupuncture is certainly an option that you should consider.

Whether acupuncture on its own can provide complete pain management or whether you need to use analgesic pharmaceuticals in combination with this particular form of natural treatment, if you can use acupuncture to reduce your pain, the level of analgesics you need will be similarly reduced.

Sometimes it is a fact that however we might prefer to use natural treatments to deal with pain, it is impractical to do so from time to time, particularly where pain is particularly extreme. In this case, painkilling drugs may well be necessary but if they can be combined with a natural solution like acupuncture to reduce the amount of drugs necessary, this helps to reduce the toxicity and therefore the potential adverse side-effects that you might be risking by taking these drugs.

CHAPTER 13- CAN HYPNOSIS RELIEVES PAIN, RELIEVES FATIGUE?

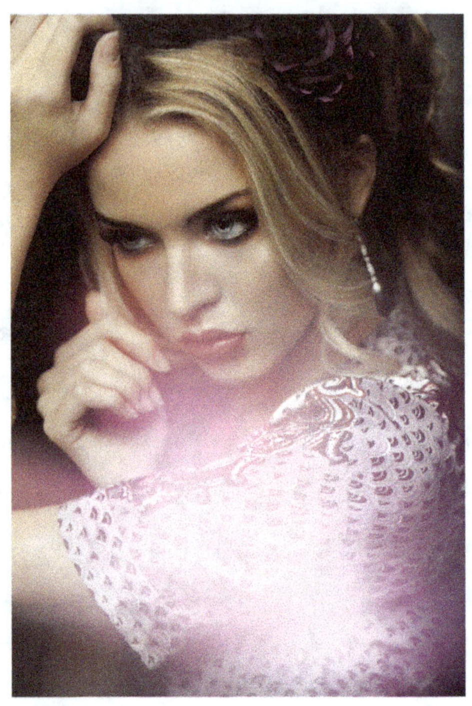

Whilst for most members of the public, hypnosis is most commonly associated with hilariously funny stage shows where people do apparently crazy things or perhaps with bad TV sitcoms, the view of the medical and psychological community of what hypnosis is all about is very different.

Indeed, since it was first invented by Franz Anton Mesmer in the 1700, it has become increasingly widely accepted that using hypnosis can deal with or 'treat' many seemingly intractable problems, including the management of chronic pain.

For a long time, the view of many medical professionals was not all that different to the view of people who watch on-stage hypnosis shows, mainly because Western medicine has always tended to assume that finding a solution to a problem always involves 'temperature-taking and shot-giving'. Hence, the idea that something as seemingly esoteric as hypnosis could play any genuine part in dealing with medical or psychological problems was simply too much for people of this nature to take on board.

But the fact is that when scientifically applied by a professionally qualified hypnotherapist, hypnosis is a remarkably effective technique that can be applied to dealing with a huge range of problems and difficulties. For example, hypnosis is often used as a highly effective way of convincing people to stop smoking whilst it is also used to treat those who genuinely want to stop drinking and others who suffer because of a similarly obsessive or addictive personality.

Most importantly, over the last 20 or 30 years, hypnosis has been subjected to the continual scrutiny of many clinical trials and in almost every situation scenario; it has been proved that hypnosis is an effective way of combating pain. People suffering from pains associated with cancer, kidney stones, gallstones, backache and invasive dental and medical procedures have all been treated or dealt with whilst under hypnosis with remarkably successful result.

According to one noted psychiatrist, Dr David Spiegl M.D. of Stanford University, 'Changing your mental set can change what's going on in your body', and all of the available evidence indicates that this is exactly right as far as dealing with chronic pain is concerned.

During the process of being hypnotized, the subject is lulled into a state of focused concentration, inner absorption plus intensely focused attention and all at exactly the same time as they are completely relaxed. Hence, because of their mental state, the subject in this pre- hypnotic state is able to pick up suggestions far more effectively than they might otherwise do in their conscious state whilst they can also tap into unused mental powers to expand the boundaries of physical possibilities.

Over the years, many papers and studies have provided compelling evidence that hypnosis is highly effective when it comes to dealing with pain.

For instance, in the April 29, 2000 edition of 'The Lancet', there was a report comparing the results enjoyed by patients under hypnosis with those under standard medical care who were undergoing invasive medical surgery. The results showed that the patients who were hypnotized suffered considerably less pain and anxiety than those who were using standard medical painkillers. In addition, the medical process itself took considerably less time to complete for the hypnotized patients, probably because there was no necessity to keep controlling their pain and calming their anxiety as there was with patients under standard anesthetic.

The final clincher was the fact that post-operation, the patients who had been hypnotized required less than half the amount of painkillers that the patients who had operated on using standard anesthetic procedures did.

This once again highlights the fact that in many cases, hypnosis is used in combination with traditional analgesic or anesthetic practices, although there is no reason why it cannot be used on its own in certain circumstances.

For instance, Dr. Alexander Levitan who is a medical oncologist in Minnesota reports that he has conducted many operations including tracheotomies and hysterectomies using nothing but hypnosis as the anesthetic.

There are many different theories as to why hypnosis would work in such a situation, with some suggesting that because hypnosis alters your expectations or perceptions of how intense the pain is going to be, this changes how you experience that pain a little later. Alternatively, another theory suggests that hypnosis focuses your attention on other objectives or images which shifts your primary focus away from concentrating on the pain.

There are many studies currently being carried out to discover exactly why hypnosis is so effective in blocking pain, many of which are focusing on the physiological changes (the changes in your brain) that take place whilst you are under hypnosis.

From these studies, it seems likely that hypnosis activates certain parts of the brain that are concerned with focusing attention. In effect, hypnosis enables your brain to focus on something completely different than the pain. In this way your brain is prevented from bringing the pain that you were previously suffering or were about to suffer to conscious awareness.

So, now you know that pain relief is 100% possible through the use of hypnosis, the next question is, what are you going to do about it?

The first option is to find a hypnotist or hypnotherapist in your neighborhood who can help you by analyzing your problems and then hypnotizing you in order to start addressing your pain.

Finding a suitable hypnotist or hypnotherapist

Before you do this, however, there are a couple of things you should do.

Firstly, you should talk to your regular doctor or medical practitioner, the person who is presently charged with keeping your pain under control. Understand that when you do so, they may not approve of what you are thinking of doing, especially as by seeking the help of a hypnotist, you are to a certain extent rebuffing their assistance.

Trust me, it is possible that your doctor will react in this way – if they have been treating even sometime, you probably know them better than most, so you may have an idea of how they are likely to react already, but it could happen.

But the fact is you are not there to ask for their approval or recommendation. What you need to know is whether subjecting yourself to hypnotism poses any real physical health risks, whether for example a pre-existing medical condition could be exacerbated by the experience.

In effect, what you are looking for is the medical all-clear so if your doctor does not approve of the idea of you seeking hypnotism for any reasons other than those which are strictly medical, it is your decision whether you choose to listen to them.

Secondly (and assuming that you decide to go ahead with trying hypnotism), you need to find a hypnotist who is capable of treating the problem that you are going to present to them. Whilst most professional hypnotists or hypnotherapists are going to be able to deal with more 'run of the mill' demands such as people who want to stop smoking and so on, not every hypnotist is going to be capable of or comfortable with the idea of dealing with chronic pain.

Consequently, you may need to contact a few appropriately qualified professionals to see whether they can help you. Pay them a visit to see whether you can get along with them, whether they are convincing when they suggest that they can help you and so on.

In short, you need to feel 100% comfortable with the hypnotist or hypnotherapist you are planning to work with because if you are not, there is an immediate element of strain or stress introduced into the relationship which is not going to help you to achieve the results that you're looking for.

The second alternative is to learn self-hypnosis. And if that sounds crazy, prepare to think again!

Can self hypnosis really work?

Can you remember the last time you went to see a movie at the cinema or movie theatre? If you can and it was a popular movie, you were probably not the only person in the cinema, just one of 200 or 300 excited souls waiting for the lights to go down so that the entertainment could begin.

When the house lights were bright, you were probably looking around, fully well aware of all of these people, but as soon as the lights went down and the movie started, you were very quickly completely engrossed (assuming that it was a good movie).

In this situation, you have effectively switched your point of focus from the real world of which we are all aware to the movie and you have done so completely. To coin a cliché, the real world has ceased to exist and the only world is that of the movie.

The principal of self hypnosis is not especially different to this basic concept. It is all about shifting and concentrating your focus, and the more successfully you can do so, the easier self-hypnosis becomes.

Most encouragingly, it is normally suggested that the ability to hypnotize yourself depends to a large extent on your desire to do so and your need to control your pain. In short, the majority of people who want to control their pain through self hypnosis manage to do so by sheer willpower and force of personality.

Having some guidance of how you can focus your attention at will is probably a useful thing, particularly at the beginning, so consulting a hypnotist or hypnotherapist who can help you to develop your own abilities is likely to be worth the effort. In this way, you get the proper guidance from the beginning and are taught by someone who really knows what they are doing.

On the other hand, there are plenty of web sites where you can learn everything you could ever need to know about self hypnosis, which has the advantage that you, can learn self hypnosis in your own time and in the comfort of your own home.

But however crazy it might sound, self hypnotism is an effective way of dealing with pain completely naturally. At the same time, because a critical part of the self hypnosis process is your ability to relax more than you have ever relaxed before, the overall benefits to your health brought about by the inevitable reduction in stress and tension this causes will be a significant boost in your battle against pain.

There is one final alternative that you might like to consider.

I have already mentioned that a Google search will pull up many results related to self hypnosis products or services being sold on the net.

Some of these products, many of which are CD or DVD presentations by professional hypnotherapists that will teach you to hypnotize yourself at home may represent an investment that is worth consideration.

Chapter 14- Herbs Naturally Relieve Pains and Fatigue

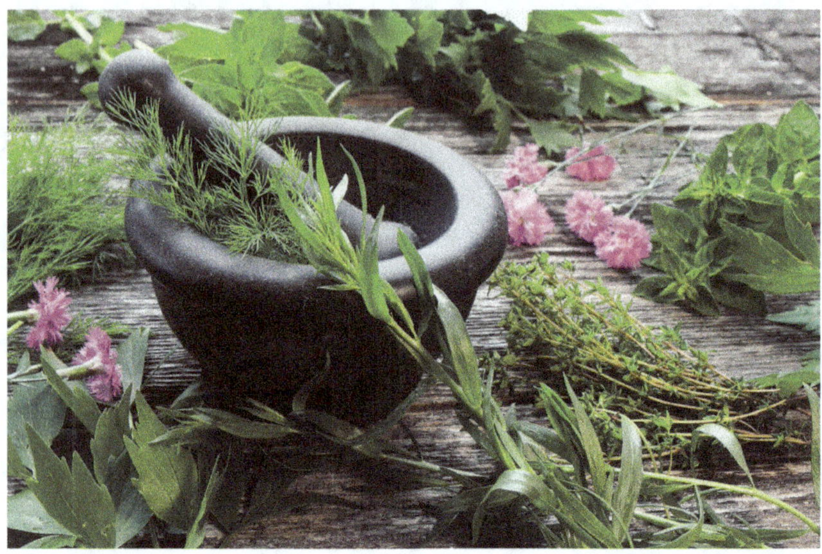

There are plenty of herbs and herbal remedies that are believed to have pain killing qualities, although it is generally accepted that most of these natural remedies are not as powerful as the pharmaceutical alternatives.

Hence, whilst the herbs and herbal treatments recommended in this section of the report will provide relief from some pains and aches, they are unlikely to be effective if you are in extreme, acute or severe chronic pain. Nevertheless, all of these remedies are worth trying if you are in some pain and want to solve the problem naturally and quickly.

Willow bark

It should perhaps be no surprise to know that willow bark is an effective herbal pain killer when you realize that the main active ingredient in aspirin (acetylsalicylic acid) is a derivative of salicylic acid which is one of the three main ingredients of the willow bark herb.

It was this connection between the active ingredient in what is still the world's most popular over-the-counter painkiller and the active ingredient in willow bark that originally suggested that it would be a successful herbal painkiller. Unfortunately however, because the absorption rate of salicylic acid from willow bark is somewhat slower than the absorption rate of its chemical cousin and because there is a longer duration, the herbal remedy is not quite as effective as the chemical version.

On the other hand, there is some evidence that a sustained dose of willow bark over a week or so will start to reduce back pain (a daily dosage of 120 to 240 mg a day is recommended), while other studies suggest that a regular dose of willow bark can help to bring some relief to those suffering osteoporosis without any noticeable side-effects.

However, this is an herb that should be avoided if you have a high level of sensitivity to aspirin or suffer peptic or gastric ulcers. Moreover, if you are susceptible to diabetes, gout or have any form of kidney or liver disease, you should not use willow bark.

Peppers

Peppers or capsicums are a common foodstuff pretty much all the world nowadays, with various varieties of peppers such as jalapenos, cayenne, chili, pimento, paprika and bird's eye chilies being available almost everywhere all the year round.

Peppers of this nature contain a substance called capsaicin and the hotter the chili that you can assume is, the more of this substance it contains. In effect, capsaicin is what gives it its heat, and it is a known fact that eating hot peppers can help to improve circulation, strengthen the nervous system and heart, relieve indigestion and increased appetite as well.

However, it is capsaicin that makes peppers interesting for someone who suffers from constant chronic pain because it is believed that this particular substance has the ability to reduce the levels of the protein that is believed to transport pain signals from the nerve endings to your brain. If the levels of this transporter protein which is known as substance P can be reduced, it stands to reason that your pain will also be reduced in a similar manner, a fact which seems to be borne out by the evidence collected so far.

For example, in clinical tests, creams containing less than one present capsaicin applied topically to a pained area have been shown to ease the pain associated with shingles and cluster headaches as well as post- amputation and post-mastectomy pain.

Taken internally, capsaicin has been seen to assist in managing various gastrointestinal problems as it stimulates the flow of digestive juices and there is some evidence that the antibacterial qualities of capsaicin can help reduce colds and infections such as flu too.

Boswellia

Boswellia is a tree that is noted for its fragrant resin and it is believed by many that frankincense (the incense mentioned in the Bible) was probably a by-product of one of the four main types of Boswellia tree.

Boswellia resin or extract has long been a staple of Ayurvedic medicine, with some evidence that it is a strong anti-inflammatory and can be used as a natural treatment for asthma as well.

Most importantly from a pain point of view, in a study of 30 patients suffering from osteoporosis of the knee, 1000 mg of Boswellia extract given over a period of eight weeks was shown to produce significant improvements when compared with the group who had been given a placebo.

In fact, the improvement was in some subjects noted to cause pain to recede by as much as 90% with an attendant increase in mobility and usage of the knee. On the other hand, no significant improvement was noted in the group using placebos.

Whilst most researchers believe that more studies need to be done before the case for Boswellia as a natural painkiller is established beyond all reasonable doubt, the results so far seem extremely encouraging.

Cherry fruits

The beneficial effects of the fruit of the sour cherry (Prunus cerasus) in humans have not been studied to any great extent so far, but the fact that the fruit contains substances that inhibit the growth of inflammatory enzymes in exactly the same way as does ibuprofen suggest that there are some pain killing possibilities here.

In addition, it is believed that sour cherries possess antioxidant qualities and that they may be effective for helping to inhibit the growth of colonic cancer and perhaps other forms of cancer as well.

Ginger

There is some evidence that including significant amounts of ginger in your diet (naturally or in the form of supplements) will help to offset the pain of osteoporosis and of course, including additional ginger in your diet has no adverse side-effects either.

In tests, it was indicated that including ginger extract in your daily diet may lower pain levels from osteoporosis by a reasonable amount whilst standing and walking and that overall levels of stiffness caused by the condition should decrease as well.

However, there is no evidence that including additional ginger in your diet is likely to reduce other forms of pain by a significant margin or improve your overall quality of life for anyone who does suffer chronic pain.

Curcumin

Curcumin is the main polyphenol ingredient that gives turmeric its yellow color and flavor. Turmeric is in turn is a member of the ginger family, which we have already seen possesses some painkilling qualities.

From the point of view of herbal medicine, curcumin has been shown to have very powerful anti-inflammatory qualities at least partially due to the fact that it is believed to contain a powerful COX-2 inhibitor. Indeed, in one study, curcumin was shown to be every bit as effective as cortisone when it came to dealing with acute inflammation whilst it was half as effective as the drug in dealing with chronic inflammation.

Given these powerful anti-inflammatory qualities, it is perhaps no surprise that curcumin has been shown to help relieve pain in conditions where inflammation is a integral factor in causing pain. Included in this list of conditions where curcumin may be able to help reduce pain are osteoporosis, ulcerative colitis, rheumatoid arthritis and fibromyalgia.

Although there are no known side effects from using curcumin as a natural painkilling treatment, it is not suitable for those who have hyperacidity problems, stomach ulcers or gallstones.

Conclusion

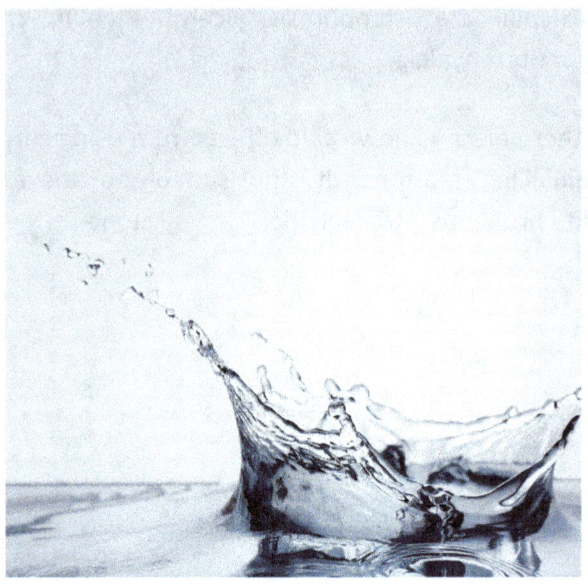

Not many people may have realized it but being enthusiastic in life gives you the power to change your life, positively. You can see things differently and give you the chance to accept and appreciate life even more. In return life will become a lot easier to live. Enthusiasm is the positive energy that drives you to reach your goal. Some people are driven by money, some by material things and by love.

These are the factors that motivate you and give you happiness in life as well as giving a whole new meaning to your existence. It is always present to everybody but only a few are able to use it for their good. Seeing everything in a positive way or allowing your mind to think that something good will turn out even after a huge blow will eventually lead you to your lifelong dream.

The most common factor that drives people to move forward is love and affection. It can be for your family, your parents, a girlfriend, a friend or for a pet. Doing everything for your loved one will give you a fire inside you that burns and let you "chug" your way up. It is a very powerful feeling that will allow you to think that everything will turn out right despite the hindrances and your limitation.

Enthusiastic people are positive people and are totally different from the rest. In the event that stressful issues and problem arises, most people would show negative signs and turn cranky, moody and grumpy. But with the enthusiastic ones, they always find a reason to smile and be happy with a tiny possibility that might eliminate the problem at hand.

If you can make yourself that person, then you are on the right track. Your most anticipated success will be nearer and you will find that life is indeed great. Planning each day enthusiastically will allow you to appreciate everything that is in front of you. You would know what you will be doing the next day and thinking ahead will provide you with ideas that can turn it into a great day.

Having an enthusiastic life is living a healthy life. You won't have to think more about problems and other concerns that will put your spirits down since your mind will permanently have a reason to cheer you up. Inspiration works and it can be anything that can motivate you. Inserting motivating activities in between your responsibilities will allow your happy thoughts keep on flowing.

Simple things like calling home and checking on your family will give you happiness. If your heart's pleasure is drinking coffee after work then look forward to it. It doesn't have to be a huge thing before you consider it special. You simply have to make it your reason for smiling and everything will fall into place. The next day will be all happy and gay if you plan it to be one. Happiness can do wonders and you can be one if you live life enthusiastically.

ABOUT THE AUTHOR

Deborah Adams noticed that the most common problem of the human society nowadays is the kind of lifestyle that we are in – very demanding, fast pace and stressful. She thinks that if we don't know how to pause and think on how to manage this in a smart way – soon stress and fatigue will swallow us whole.

That is why Deborah put all her resources to gather all the information needed to better understand on how we can fight chronic fatigue.

Deborah is living in Kansas with her husband.